NOT YET:

A care-giving collage

Dear Barbara,

How many years?
Near 50! It's
soon our golden
anniversary! Long
may it continue!
Love to you,
Marcia

ALSO BY MARCIA SLATKIN

NOT YET:

A Care-Giving Collage

A Healing Journey
through
Alzheimer's Care-Giving

by

MARCIA SLATKIN

STEPHEN F. AUSTIN STATE UNIVERSITY PRESS
2012

Stephen F. Austin State University Press
P.O. Box 13007, SFA Station
Nacogdoches, TX 75962-3007
sfapress@sfasu.edu

Cover image: Doris Smilowitz, by Arthur Silk, www.silkphoto.com
Book Design: Laura McKinney, Brittany O'Sullivan

LIBRARY OF CONGRESS IN PUBLICATION DATA
Slatkin, Marcia
Not Yet: A Care-Giving Collage
p. cm.
ISBN: 978-1-936205-49-3

1. Poetry 2. American Poetry 3. Alzheimer's Disease 4. Care-Giving
5. Slatkin, Marcia

The paper in this book meets the requirements of ANSI / NISO
Z39.48-1992 (R1997) (Permanence of Paper)

To Doris (Dora) Smilowitz, paragon of initiative, hard work and encouragement.

To my devoted siblings and their spouses: Jessica and Jeff Pearson, Henry and Connie Smilowitz, Pat Rosso /Robert Smilowitz.

To Doris's ten grandchildren, all care-givers in unique ways.

To Dan, who hung in while I ministered to Doris, even though I sorely neglected him.

To magically spiritual Leah, who at the very end, held, sang to, and eased our mother into whatever follows.

Additional Praise for Not Yet

In luminous lines, each page a small, lush painting, Slatkin's work respects the person within the patient, forgives the sins of the past, sees the possibility for wholeness within diminishment, and finds the 'peace of closeness' in any moment of intimacy. Every caregiver, every family member, every poet should read these poems. Those who do will be humbled and changed.

> —Cortney Davis, poet, *Body Flute*, *Details of Flesh*, *Leopold's Maneuvers*

An unflinching observer, Slatkin allows herself honesty mixed with tenderness, a triumph over pathos.

> —Claire Nicolas White, author, *Death of the Orange Trees*, editor, *Oberon Poetry Review*

The poems are honest, raw, close to the heart. They will speak to, console, and inspire you.

> —Phillip Levine, actor, poetry editor *Chronogram*

This insightful book carefully preserves the humanity and basic dignity of both caregivers and those diagnosed with Alzheimer's Disease. The poems come alive, and their wide range of emotions will both touch your heart, and offer hope and encouragement.

> —Ethel M. Thomas, Qualified Dementia Care Specialist

Acknowledgments

The following poems, "The Loss," "Home," "The Fluorescent Bulb," "Solicitude," "A Late Blessing," "the Bath," "The Achievement," "Intellectual Opiate," "Aquaria," "Pedicure," "The Right Scooping Spoon," "The Trip," " Wonder Land," "The Thigh's Mind," "The Garden," "Life Lines," "Family Pressure," "Personality Intact," "Thrills," and "At Least This," were all published in *I Kidnap My Mother*, Finishing Line Press, 2005.

"Solicitude" won "best poem" in the *Contexts* Magazine Contest, Stony Brook Medical School, 2005, and was published there.

"Devolution" was published in *Long Island Sounds Anthology*, June 2007

"Gregor Samsa's Sister" was published in the Summer 2007 issue of *Oberon*.

"Repairs" was published in *Crone* magazine, 2008.

"Mummies: Guanajuato, Mexico" was published by *Calyx* magazine, Jan 2009.

"A Late Blessing" is part of an anthology called *AFTER SHOCKS, The Poetry of Recovery*, edited by Tom Lombardo, 2008.

Six poems, "My Hollowed Mother," "Shift / Change," "That Home Song and Dance," "The Need For Mother," "Being of Use," and "Toileting" were published by *Ars Medica*, Mt Sinai Hospital, Toronto School of Medicine, Ontario, Canada, 2008.

"Mother's Day" was published by the Performance Poet's Association's Twelfth Annual Literary Review, *PPA LR #12*, Summer 2008

"Teaching" was published in the *Long Island Sounds Anthology*, 2008.

"Roles Reversed" was published by the *Long Islander*, Huntington, NY, Nov, 2009

"The Gates," *Xanadu* magazine, 2011.

"Not Yet," poem, a finalist in the *Naugatuck River Review*'s narrative poetry contest, published Winter 2011.

"Apology," "The Gambler" were published in *LIFEBLOOD*, Chickaree Press, 2011.

"My Brother Cares for our Mother" was published in *Chronogram*, March 2011.

Contents

2005

2006

2007

Birthday--1994

This year, her card
comes as usual, but
the script is jagged,
the loops veer,
the "O"s are wavering lines
thick with trying to steer
impossible curves. She says
kind things, there is
a check, and an old photo.

Small, stained, it came
from my father's wallet
forty years ago -- shrubs
blotched, lawn-space wholly
faded. We are in a park,
my youngest siblings not yet born,
one brother on his knees,
hair mussed, a grumpy bear.
I scrunch my first-grade chest.
My mother's features blear.

My father, now dead twenty
years, seems calm – no hint of wit
or sudden flash-flood rage.
You can't discern a mustache,
or the cow-lick riots
within his thick red mane.
And see? His whole right side
is bleached, and blends
with grass that fades toward
blurred, formless trees.

"I hope," my mother writes
on the card's blank half,
"that nothing I am sending
makes you sad."

Apology

While giving care,
I search for gestures
that reveal;
the telling quote,

my mother unaware
that I sift our days,
and frame a farce
of confusion, a lyric
taming fear – then pool
our pain to write
a one-act play.

Dear God, forgive
this use. Taught
to not waste time,
I harbor an urge
to weave words
as deep as the need
to calm an itch.
This pool of subject,
angst and muse
is a gift I accept.

And the love
I bear this woman,
despite myself,
is deep, and perhaps
evident

2004

The Loss

In her space,
no surface was clear.

Stained, mended,
they lay everywhere,
only the kitchen
free of piles
heaped for decades
from *thrifts* so cheap,
her wallet felt heavier
after a purchase
than before she paid.

For hours, she'd refold,
move stacks to new corners,
hide things she feared
the super desired
for his wife.

When I drugged,
then stole her,
the small suitcase
stunned.

And now, though I promise
her troves wait in Brooklyn,
she camps near my alien
closet. Bereft,
she rifles through, sorts,
mourns, then sifts

shards of her mind
for an image
of her treasure gone.

Home

When her pills can't fill in blanks,
follow dots, cover rage with calm,
she cries for home –

fights to be there, sure
she can manage alone,
unaware that tangled clumps

       block streets between lights--
       strike coordinates of space
       and time; of goal and how to
       get to; erase recent events
       and how things connect –
       hiding all in plumes
       tangled as fleece,
       or the sticky comb of bees.

So home is the kingdom of *can*
that was cruelly taken --
that should still be, and *would*
materialize, if we'd just let her
go there and try – let her
fling wide the doors and find,
grab, embrace
all that waits
to fill her open hand,
her groping mind.

The Fluorescent Bulb

flickers, part able to glow
weakly, the rest rust-brown
which slowly fades to gray.

Ten times an evening
I'll forget, and hit the switch
for the light I've always known,
each time surprised
by absence, noting
the effort – a fit, a start,
a sputtering stab at function,
while I pray
that this time wires
connect—

like looking at my mother
now, and craving
bridges to span
billions of gaps.

Solicitude

Amid a maze
of age spots, raised
as gravel, walnut hued
and jagged in shape,

my mother's breasts
emerge, still pink,
unscarred though fallen,
guileless on a sheet
of rippled skin.

And after donning
bra and snapping
straps in place,
she gathers them up

        like scooping pliant
        honey with a spoon,
        or shaping dough
        to buns that fit a pan--

and rests
obedient lobes
in waiting slings
slowly -- cradling each
with vein-rich
careful hands.

Lacking Matrix

Liebnitz knew.
In the absence of functioning mind,
all incoming colors, textures, sounds
are dots by Seurat which,
wrenched out of canvass,
are strewn to the wind, links
splintered, then randomly lumped.

While those without ears, or born blind,
lack data, thus nose through the air,
bump into trees, scrape perilous rocks
in the deep, or tunnel with moles,

the sensate Alzheimer's mind
can collect but not sort,
can observe, not connect,
and will always,
always forget.

The Seeds of Disease

Suspecting allergy,
we stop her new meds,
and after a day my mother rages.
She is a writhing spider,
all legs in pain. Pacing,
each step bears exclamation
point weight, each glare, anger
in italicized caps. I am the enemy
she wants to escape, Brooklyn
once again the promised land.

What then is real?
Does it *all* boil down
to chemistry? Is there
nothing more innate?

What of childhood fights --
nights of hiccupping sobs
on my bed as I gulped back
wrath, abandoned protest,
and longed to be held, loved?
Was that chemistry? Hers
or mine? And this raging
mother so reminiscent
of life in times bygone –

were the seeds of disease
soaking, secretly
swelling even then?

A Late Blessing

I wake her with touch,
rubbing her shoulders,
saying the time.

With a hug, I bend
toward the arc
of her chest. My arms
encircle, my side
hugs her length.

Near the sink,
I reach for the kettle
by nudging her cheek
with my forehead.
I snuggle, then smile
at her squeal.
Despite her greased
face at sleep time,
I kiss her, wish her
good dreams.

This is the mother I battled
when young, the mother
who beat my defiance;
the one I hit back

While we walk now,
she proffers her hand,
its gnarled back spotted –
but its guileless palm
soft as a persimmon,
trusting as a child.

The Bath

Bonnard was right.

Not as she stands to dry,
shoulders bent, ribs wide,
spine a ridged bow;

nor as she turns to dress,
her buttocks flaccid
as last year's peaches
kept cold, skin creased
to soft folds.

Yet when she lies immersed,
her compact form is winsome,
ironed to smoothness,
colors blurred and deeply drenched.

Bonnard knew that a woman
afloat in a tub is an icon,
serene and open
even near ninety,
alive in liquid
blue and yellow light.

Intellectual Opiate

My mother listens
to tapes in the car –
Cogito ergo, Descartes,
optics, psychology,
and when I offer music
instead, or local news,
she stays my hand,
mesmerized by words
she does not understand
but finds sublime.

       "He said
Psychology. I got
my masters from Columbia,"
she says. "I studied that."

Eyes closed, she sinks
to a satisfied trance,
protected by culture
she deems fitting,
not small-town or crass;
lulled by thoughts
that ... transcend.

Aquaria

Do not look to the writhing
octopus, or the darting,
eel. Do not admire the flitting
angel fish, the lively tang,
the lyretail. Consider instead

the red pacu: huge, placid,
merely floating,
slow eyes unperturbed.

Do you expect more of that fish
than his being alive, suspended
without evident curiosity?

All life is blessed,
even when diminished,
even when changed
so only drops
of the past remain.

I show the fish
to my mother,
and she nods.

Entanglement

We walk in woods
near a school. The trees
have not yet leafed,
it is a brisk, clear day
in early spring.
But my mother is afraid.

"How far?"
she wants to know.
"Have we started
back? Will we
find our way?"

And even in near
sight, she can't see
structure through a forest
dense as mind.

I think thick branches
weave behind her eyes
even as we touch
car doors, she grateful
she's survived
the wild.

Pedicure

After her soak,
I note her toenails—
spikes, tapers, cones, a mattock,
duck beaks, a scythe.

Even more strange
is the thick gum beneath --
white paste that I rub
from under and between.
Crusts mass like crushed
shell, pile like scree.

I clip all easily now,
and expect that,
when she rises,
my mother will lift - off
and fly, cast free –

her feet light
as helium balloons,
                    or sunrise.

At the Center--The Achievement

We are late.
Breakfast plates are stacked
for washing, chairs set
for exercise with weights.

I watch my mother take a seat,
straight in her chair, eager
to confront this day with elders
demented to varying degrees. The leader

sings out the week's programs
for my sake: a Christmas party,
visits from the children,
baking, singing, pictionary, crafts.

I am brought to see
last Friday's work now hardened,
each piece labeled, and I look
for my mother's name, Doris,
searching 12 wreaths in vain,
my heart sinking, then finally
find hers -- number 13. It,

like the others, is dark
green, with red poinsettias
round the plaster pine,
and as I start to exclaim, to praise
this achievement, my nose suddenly
stings, my eyes fill, voice turned liquid.
Fighting for a hearty pitch, I say,
"mama, what a lovely wreath!",
                    then throw a kiss,
                    and leave her to enjoy the day.

The Pageant We Are Part of

The center gleams The staff.
wear hats, all is red
and green, volunteers
play piano, sing.

Both elders and guests
follow song sheets,
strike bells and chant
as staff aid the dance,

and my rosy-cheeked mother
is entranced by this cloak
of tinsel and kindness,
mirror and smoke.

So we serve one another.
Those with strong hands
do crochet or Chopin
for friend or for family.
We fold love into touch,

and rub honey on toast
for slow eaters
who need to be coaxed.

The Trip

Slowly, we move
toward the covered canal
leading planeward,
till I'm told I can't
go further.

I show my mother
the photo of my sister
pinned to her blouse,
I name family members
she will visit,

but she feels betrayed.
As an attendant
wheels her away,
the spokes weave
a growing web of distance,
and she cries my name,

her soul steeped in fear
so thick it dissolves
identity, and what, at journey's
end, she'll find.

Maybe that's how it will
finally be for most – unable
to fathom destination,
or believe that others wait
on another side.

Wonder Land

A diligent host,
my sister cuts my mother's
dose, saying exercise
and distraction
mitigate psychosis.

My mother is a strong
swimmer, yet I dream
of her barely treading water,
nose bobbing just above

the waves. My sister
will pull her past rapids,
through torrents,
away from breakers,
but might not see
a surge, a rippling
swell, the splash
that stings and causes
heavy breathing.

In the dream, my mother
is Alice, swimming
with the door mouse
in a pool of tears.
My mother's tears?
Or perhaps mine?
Maybe it is I
who need treatment,
and the smaller
dose is fine.

Milk and Meat

In the next room,
my mother speaks
of her life as a Jew –

> "My parents were orthodox."
> They prayed, went to *shul*
> on *Shabos* – but mainly,
> milk and meat were separated –
> two sets of dishes, silver,
> towels --all different.

> "But when I searched in biology,
> chemistry, nutrition -- there was
> no scientific basis."

When I enter, I speak
of Deuteronomy,
where it is forbidden to boil
a kid in its mother's milk.
"That's the real reason,"
I explain. "The sages
were humane."

But because of her age,
I don't speak of times
I felt singed by the flames
of her rage.

Family Pressure

"Less is more
when it comes to meds"
my brother says.
"I did it on less,"
says my sister.
"Just… try."

    At first
I lie, then comply.
But mom seems a rat
in a maze, on a trial
to withhold needed food.

She grunts with each breath.
Her questions are machine-guns
fired at forgotten events.
Her stomach aches, she looses
track and trace, weeps,
and accuses me! Our moist
salve of laughter dries,
leaving bald places.

So I increase.
The rat escapes the cage.
Winter spins to spring.
With some meds,
less is … less.

In Retrospect...

At first, my house was wilderness,
and her Brooklyn center shone.
They had world-events there,
classes on art, and hundreds
of young folk.

But in focused moments
my mother looks back.

"It was lonely," she says.
"People at the center
were all paired with friends
or as part of a group.
I was an alien, an outcast –
so I just sat. This center

is better. We all talk
to staff. Then, I have you
to be with at night. I had
nothing to do, home, alone
in the evenings. I don't want
to go back."

At Least This

I stoop
to pull the diaper
up around my mother's
waist, my temple
near her breasts,
and feel soft palms
caress my head, frail
arms enfold my neck.

It is fields near Arles
ablaze with sun-lit poppies;
the musk of haystacks
dried in August heat.
It is simmered milk
in mugs that heat
numb hands; the pregnant
flame of buds in early
spring. It's the peace

of closeness – no matter
what else comes.

2005

Care-Giving

Our fights now distant
past, we are two women
often home alone.

My mother's modesty
dissolves as I button and zip.

After meals, I monitor her pills,
mindful of the blue one
that brings peace.

I joke, repeat, plan calming
tasks. We walk slowly holding hands
on local streets. At night, I bathe her clean.
If still fertile, I think
we'd bleed at the same hour.

And yet, she treasures one son
more. Her skin flushes as they speak,
open as an iris, lush, alive.

And with my sister,
food-talk is robust.

But if our love
wells for seconds,
fleeting as the honeysuckle
strains of a mid-spring breeze
inhaled deeply--
that is enough.

Repairs

If my mother were a cello
I'd rescued from an attic,
strings loose, bridge
warped, seams un-
glued, sound post
clawed by beetles,

I'd do repairs --
as I have tools to plumb
and probe, aged maple,
heat enough to steam the bridge
and set it straight, a way
to patch cracks carefully,
with unctuous glue and clamps,
which I can use to attach a bar
below the "C." I'd cut and fit
a post between belly
and back – then unwrap

new strings. Weighing
gut or steel, I'd choose
Jargar for long wear.

Tuners would be next.
I'd slowly
      bring her
                up
                      to pitch

until the fifths were true,
then varnish her belly
russet and gold. Though sick

and old, I'm sure
she'd be less bent,
her mind more sane,
her burnished frame
more fit to play
the insistent pulse
and fervor of her soul.

The Gates

After an article on "Christo Gates"
NY Times, February 13, 2005

When my brother sends
an e-mail on the "Christo
Gates," large font,

I print it, paste
photos of the park
on back, and give
the whole to mom,
saying "Bobby sent it."

Since it's from him,
she holds it with her
all that day, up to
the light, enlarging
text with a glass
and repeating phrases
that to her make sense:

"You have 16 days,"
she reads. *"Don't delay."*
And later, *"Be fore-warned,"*
she intones, so I hear
and almost see
the gates -- not pearly,
but a creamy orange-gold.

"They're warning us,"
she explains. *"Time is
fleeting."*

Life Lines

Sometimes she will panic,
trapped in quicksand
and treading, eyes
veiled, nose covered,
arms groping, desperate
for a freeing rope.

And she is grateful
that I cast my coiled
cable, thick with news
of family she can grab.

As she holds the line,
pinched shoulders go slack.
The vessels of her face
dilate. Eyes focused, face
flushed, relaxed, she studies
photos. Loved ones

crowd the void as she cradles
braided context,
thrust into the world again,
a person with a life.

At the Senior Center

It is almost four. Elders
rise, jacks in a box erupting
at different times, pacing,
tugging on coats,
lurching toward glass
to glimpse a pick up,
begging to escape.

Only my mother sits,
an oasis of concentration,
intent on plastic letters
which she crafts to meaning,
a shiny Buddha
with a smiling face.

When I come near
and kiss her cheek,
she smiles contentedly.
"Look at all the words
I made," she says.

The Right Spoon

You can reach in
and scoop out the good parts.

Though dry seeds
fill much of the whole,
and chatter as cold teeth
at myriad ills,

with soft shoe or touch ,
a clown smile or skin-rubbing hug,
you can free pulp from dread,
surround and encase it --

so both of you savor
wet flesh of papaya or melon,
sweet through and through.

You harvest best focus and fun
by choosing a well-hewn, varied,
bright scooping spoon.

The Thigh's Mind

At the gym,
my mother loves
rhythmicity -- pounding
that dogged half mile,
pulling that oar,
struggling
into machines and pushing back.

Strangers greet her,
smile, cluck about age,
offer to teach free weights.

Ruddy cheeked, eyes bright,
her hands tremble less,
and her thighs, thick
with tennis memory,
basket recall, the triumph
of ropes once climbed—

> her thighs
> hold her history,
> they her best mind.

The Garden

We talk, and my mother
walks the path of her life
as though a garden, relishing
shade her children provide,
each tree different,
productive despite scars.
She stops to touch a leaf,
notice a bloom, mourn
the blight of a sickened bud,

then stoops to weep
over the bush that was my father.
"I should have tended
you better," she whispers,
cradling roses, brown
but faintly sweet. "I should
have given you more time.
I was ambitious, selfish.
I let you die."

Her mourning wets the earth
beneath sere branches,
gnarled stem. I don't know
if tears fill some reservoir
from which my father
can still drink. But crying
seems to clear my mother's heart.

She smiles, inhales.
And at this moment,
    the walk, the garden,
    the thorny bush with thin,
    dry hips, all past perhaps
    pried free,

she seems wholly alive.

Personality Intact

My mother loves
slapstick, cackles
at Chaplin's walk,
the pregnant man's
fat-bellied waddle,
Buster Keaton's
mournful panic -- even

her own pratfalls –
a hard sit on the toilet,
the rocking it now takes
to rise, rubbed-in toothpaste
that turns her face blue
when taken for sunblock,
though it burns
as she endures a scrub.

So, despite humiliation
or pain, my mother's
love of the absurd
keeps me sane.

Losses

Hands wringing, my mother weeps
as we search near the sink,
under sheets, in the space
beneath things. "I know

what happened," she says
as we rest, tired
of stirring dust
in this Braille
of desperate quests.

"At the Senior Center, a man
beside me touched my hand.
At first I pulled away.
Then he began to rub
each finger. It was just
a silly game…"

She demonstrates
with long, slow strokes.
"You see?" she says,
feeling her own gnarled flesh,
each tender, rhythmic caress
an evident pleasure. "Maybe
he took it then. I was
dumb to let him."

Yet tears and kneading
both have purged
her pain. Refreshed,
she seems to forget all—
her marriage, the past,
and this sad
golden theft.

Thrills

On the phone with my siblings,
our mother knocks on wood
at each grandchild's
achievement. Clutching
her chest, she begs all
to watch out, take care, be safe.

But when in our car
we dart down a hill,
she gasps as the land
sweeps toward her.
The pitch into space
mimics the pulse of flight.
"I love it rushing up,"
she confides. "It wakes me."

And when my husband drives,
she squeals with delight
at speed. "It's good when
you go fast" she cries,
gripping his arm, the big
man she reveres.
"It's so exciting."

"Don't tell anyone," he warns,
"or I'll get in trouble."

"I won't," she says,
conspiratorial to the core.
Then, "Go fast again." she begs.

Awareness

They say
its mercy is oblivion.
The ill are not aware
of all they lack..

But when my mother hears
of past events, she rages,
her memories crushed
by vengeful teeth
that grind treasure.

At other times,
she shrugs and blames
old age.

At our *seder,*
the *haroset* was pungent
and sweet, the ritual
streamlined. When
we got to the story
of the four sons,
she stared at me,
and tried to speak.

Later, when it came time
for the youngest child to hide
the *afikomen*, she volunteered.

"I'll be the simple son," she cried,
grabbing the *matzo,* laughing.

Mother's Day

causes pieces
heaped in her mind
to yearn for wholeness.
Her questions are urgent;
impatient as horse-tails
swatting flies.
"Are you my daughter"?

she asks, stern, wanting the issue
finally settled. When I say
"Yes," she asks if this
was true long ago.

Craving clarity
about the father of my siblings,
she is shocked that theirs
is also mine. Rummaging
through the past, "Wasn't there
a divorce?" she asks.
When I insist her marriage
stayed whole, she is relieved.

So we migrate to authority:
the arbiter of blood lines,
incontrovertible evidence
of relationships –
the chart full of photos
on her wall. Puzzle
complete, the family
is spread, a royal
flush with her face
the heart-brimming queen
in its center, beaming.

Skipping Bones

For my mother, the earth
oozes. Fears bubble up
from marshes where monsters,
caught at the bottom, rot.

She's adept. Once
she's smelled them,
she'll put hand in and scoop,
then skip their bones over slime.

She gets twenty jumps to a throw,
each bone spun with vigor
enough to keep panic aloft
indefinitely, till I break

the trance, wake her with food,
hugs, games -- then march her
far from the tarn of malaise
into sun -- and smile,

hiding from her what I know
about real bones with which
men litter the world.

Indeed, the ground we walk on
hides pain wanton and deadly
as any delusion.

Media distracts as though
I were senile too. So I read
between, hear around, see through

and learn of stones spewing fire,
rocks oozing gall, boulders
that quake and bleed,
which powerful men
aim at city, sand and sea
daily, without end.

From this
there is no waking.

Potency--An Ode to Geodon

I can't imagine
what it must do,
forcing its way through
the curd that clogs
my mother's brain.

But after a dose, her fists
no longer clench and pound.
Her jaw less set, skin
less taut, the abyss
blurs, grows distant.

Can the capsule's powder
devour the plaque?
Does it sweep filth away,
or sniff it out? Is it
a sucking action?
Or perhaps it explodes
waste, a suicide bomber
then itself lost
within the toxic gel --

for any of which
I am grateful.

Devolution

A girl
holds her parent's wrist.

Swaddled in maternal arms,
an infant, head bobbing,
burrows in deeply,
a hibernating cub.

These days, my mother's hand
slides into mine: pliant,
dappled as banana skin
warmed by sun. Her grip fits.
We walk everywhere this way --
through the house, out to the bus,
toward the treadmills at the gym.

But I accept what's to come.
Soon, only hugs
will nourish.

Break Through

Care-giving can be
custodial – lotion
on toes before socks,
a brisk wash,
 a kiss on the cheek.

But sometimes,
her heart-shaped face
held between my palms,
her eyes locked deeply
into mine, care is transmuted
as coal to diamonds
under love's pressure.

So, air no longer
warm, the gardener,
faced with last year's
grey, sere stalks,
begins to pull
what must be cleared.

But look! Beneath
dry clumps he finds
rich soil. Hands work
this earth, and inspire,
through time, the open
lips of iris, the poppy's
deepest eye.

At Every Level

When at last I find my mother,
the woman beside her
begins to sing, as a thrush
fills the air with robust trill.

"She is so smart, so
caring, such a pleasure
to be with," this woman cries.

So I smile, grateful
that even at ninety,
amid the severely demented,
there wells the same
hearty pleasure
I know when, gaining
a new friend,
we dive into talk
that excites.

What She Wants

She had just
found him again, this absent
son she loved. She had just
realized who, pushed plug
through socket. Juice
lit her face,

and then, he left.
I cooked, thinking
all was tidy, tucked
shut, we could
go on. But she wouldn't
begin. "No," she said

again and again. "I'll
wait. *Tsuzammen.*
We'll eat together."

And I could see
a warm, grey tabby
on her side, four kittens
suckling opulent teats,

or a mallard
glowing green
with love of ducklings,
whom she carefully
keeps in line as they waddle
behind her, quacking.

Mummies: Guanajuato, Mexico

Clad in jackets
frayed by soil or bug
till only lining covers frame,
some still have hair – beards
or braids that curve beyond
the folds of breast turned stone.

But bones themselves remains unique--
the mottled shapes of skulls; the sink
and gape of brows and nose; the tilt
jaws took in death; the teeth.

And how did each
enfold life's sudden
end? Some hands
rest on chests in prayer;
some tightly grip a scapula.
Each mummy is a map to read.
The deepest tales stay etched.

Through glass, past years,
what's left to do
but bless each death,

then go back home
to one who sleeps --
lips pink, hands
warm atop the sheet --

the mother I can touch,
embrace --and mercifully
still kiss awake.

Massaging My Mother

The masseuse
kneads her skin
as waves carve the sand
on a beach, pulling out
and away, then back
round the scapula,

circling the discs
of her spine
the way streams
mould the silt
in their beds,
sliding stones,
sweeping rocks

like age spots
that shift beneath
fingers that circle
and press to release
　　(with a sigh, as air
　　　flows from her chest)

as rivers from heights
fall past boulders
toward rippling
peace.

Full Circle

Wherever I went
in the world –
        a store on Boul Mich,
        a museum in Munich,
        the Strand, NY, brimming
        Rockwell prints –
I'd desire bright pages,
my mind devouring
hue, form, stroke,
yet I'd feel ashamed –
there were libraries, after all;
I didn't need them.

Now, as my mother's
eyes redden and tear
when she reads,
I show her books
I bought then--
art she reveres:
Lucien Freud, Paul
Gauguin, Egon Schiele.

Hands resting on bodies entwined,
she strokes the satin limbs,
flesh fed by color and brush.
Her fingers linger
slowly as a lover would,

and touch beauty
after dinner, before bed.

Plateau

We are at a clear place now.

As when you hike
a mountain, and the rocks
are steep, their edges
sharp, the bits of clay
between them slick
with last night's rain
so that you slip
and almost fall,

but after hours
of upward climb,
the sun a weight
atop your head,
you come upon
a grassy place
where you can stop,
eat trail mix, drink
the water in your pack,
and rest. So with

my mother. Now
we smile, cuddle,
hug, and I --
no longer rent
by care-confines,
am somehow grown content.

2006

Roles Reversed

When I felt sick
and tired of feeling sad,
I wept. My mother
straightened her bent
back and held me,
stroked my hair,
murmuring words

like moss in woods,
honey on the tongue.

When young,
my tears came most
from wars between us.
There was no comfort.

Now she is old,
adrift in time,
plagued by fear,
needing my care,
yet can summon warmth
from some sweet well
that might have
always been there.

I heard her praise,
felt her love, and cried
luxuriantly --

her child again.

Postpartum Depression

At first,
my survey of her mal-
orientation, emaciation, illness –
was wildly compelling.
She needed medical consults,
massive supplementation,
a cornucopia of medication.

Now, my mother,
round as a panda,
sleek as an eel, is stable,
able to continue for years.

The hard work
done, the routine set,
why do our days seem
flat to me, our dealings
bleached, dusk leached
to a nondescript hue:
mere layers of gray?

Gone are the zany
quirks of her illness
that needed heroics;
gone the rhythm
of discovery and fixing.

So *drama* dissolves
to *staying power* --
a kind, upbeat smile
as through plodding years
she quietly thrives.

In My Mother's Bath

My arm cramps
as it travels the knobs
of her spine. She demands
soap, more pressure
and scrub, but I tire.
As I rub,

she wants it done
harder. I scour,
I scrape, I abrade,

then remember how others
have worked: those scything grain
through dusk; or those
who flay fish, hands
plated with silver that stinks;
those rubbing clothes
on stone in cold streams;
or those who pound corn
against rock
so their children
can eat.

The Show Must Go on

There's a rope I must ride on --
yellow, with feathers,
sparkles, balloons,

and there are gales
that dislodge me from it;
storms that tear down –

      my mother's complaints,
      or the quavering fear
      from the pit of her stomach
      that seeps into mine.

My impatience is rough
as a blast from the north,
or a cyclone's swift gust.

It grows hard to balance
on a fine beam of sweetness,
or cycle a bar above rage.

I must stop, breathe slowly,
quell squalls that startle,
quench slow burning, smoke-
spewing fire—

and remember
to always
    be kind.

A Prayer to the Dial Tone

Eyes tightly closed, holding
the buzzing phone to her heart
like a crucifix,
thumbing random numbers
like worry beads -- or perhaps
davening, as she'd doubtless
seen her father do, swaying
with each fervent phrase
whispered into the top
of the plastic messenger
of contact and warning,
my mother communicates
with the spirit of her son,
whose work entails travel:

"My sweetheart,
be safe."

The Mother and the Ticking Clock

Her call can be faint
as a thin stream of breeze
on an almost still night;
the sound of her rising
quiet as a plate
so subtly embossed,
raised and flat
seem the same;

yet I hear her-- a sigh
pierces doors, a grunt
hits my ear as dire need.

And when I am deep
in thought, even asleep,
her voice seeps,
a trickle of cold
which chills heat in a tub;
water on water,
for a breath-beat
distinct.

When my babies were small,
my ears weren't so pealed.
I knew they were safe.

But now, I must calm her,
hear the complaints
which then melt,
like dry ice,
without trace.

Dear God, I don't mind.
But I pray that you weigh
the hours that drip
through these difficult days,
so that when, at her end,
I am free, you can refill
the cup of my life
with more time.

Memories of a Mozart March

We hear music
I learned when young.

Suddenly my mother begins
to sing, her voice
outlining the tune,
the pitches cracked
as the shell of a struck egg,
its tonal plates
set at strange degrees,
yet stuck to the skin
that gives it form.

I hear, then see
in the faltering sound
guided by that membrane,
a way in, beneath the song
itself, all the way back

to the yolk of her past.
She recalls our old
house, my piano,
and tries to stretch toward,
grope for, reach and hold

        some round,
          clear note
             that for the moment
                makes her whole.

I Know about Grief

for vanished things: the spasm.
in the stomach when your purse
disappears; the reach for rosin
that isn't there, the bow
tight with anticipation;
that piece of gum
your jaw aches to mash
now missing.

But with my mother,
the track cut by loss is deeper
than reason can fill. Put
the Vaseline jar she misplaced
before her, and she will continue
to count it gone, the thing in your hand
a mirage. Show her the toothbrush,
she'll say hers was different—
broader, larger, thicker --
she can't explain,
except that hers is lost.

She will be desolate
for hours, days, even as she uses
the disappeared cream,
even as the missing floss
slides between her teeth,
even as I grab her throat,
ready to squeeze.

No Good Deed Goes Unpunished

The need to thank
comes upon her suddenly,
like a viral attack
in the gut, or fullness
after several pots of tea.

My mother will seize my arm
and beg that I phone
my sister, who sent her
sneakers she can wear
without pain. It does

no good to explain
she has already thanked
forty times, as each word
vanished
when said. Every
step she treads
creates the need
to thank anew.

Her feet well- shod,
there will be no end.

Teaching

It is not
that different.
I a crazed
Lady Macbeth
in a nightgown,
before rapt students,
candle in hand,
and rubbing fingers stained with blood,

or playing Medea,
milking pain, letting
all the loss of my youth
bubble up through my chest
as I wail the murder
of her sons.

So with my mother
I dramatize what is:
arms raised to greet
the wind's caress,
nostrils flared
to make her really *see*
the siren rose,
to be aware, to link
sense and heart and mind --

my eyes closed, my head
thrown back to enact
the soak of the sun
by our pale, hungry skin.

My Hollowed Mother

Though ill,
for years she seemed
thick, buttery,
her colors vibrant
as squash on the vine.

All the while,
pills hid changes –
masked shrivel,
covered rot.

Fearing truth,
at each hint
of softening
I'd give more.

It's now such a time--
a breath before increase,
her shrunken contour
a gourd speckled
with mold.

When I lift, she feels light,
almost empty, her speech
a scattered moth's flight.

Quavering,
she turns to ask
if it "will be all right."

My Brother Cares for Our Mother

Despite myriad work sites
flung as a deck of cards
cut, shuffled, and strewn
a half-globe away,
he phones nightly,
his speech gentle,
his discourse jaunty
yet measured as the ticking
of a clock. Most times

they discuss the rabbit.
It runs, it sits, it eats.
It is the web he weaves
to support her, his silk
strong as steel, she
delighted to be caught
in its circular threads.

"He must be the luckiest
bunny alive," says my mother
as she smiles herself to sleep.

Grooming

At an earlier
stage of her disease,
my mother would sit in the bath
and tear at them: brown
raised cankers which,
though present for decades
and medically harmless,
now repelled her.
She'd pick them
till they bled.

When I gave her mega-
vitamin C, the cankers
thinned, flattened,
faded.

As they lost color,
I could fleck them off
like bits of glue
on skin, food
dried to a bib, or candy
stuck to a child's lip.

It has become
my obsession:
to give more "C"
and pick her clean
as though she were
a prized hen

plucked for some
glorious feast—
and not for a blank sheet
addressed to a grave.

Pleasure

Even when she wanders,
unfocused, unwilling
to chop, stir, dry,
the smells of dinner
are trumpet and flute
to my mother's blood.

Her plate seeped in siren scents,
heaped with color,
eagerness softens her face,
opens, swells it with longing --
the glow and greed
of a hungry child.

Then it is
that I remember my dog,
dear as she was to me,
and how she loved food,
would pant for it,
the one (by the end)
unambiguous pleasure,
even when tumors
made eating a chore,
even then, the life-giving
smell, the juice
and crunch of it
was (besides
petting, perhaps)
the best consolation.

Gregor Samsa's Sister

I try not to think of her
after his death -- opening
windows to air the bedding,
stretching her young arms
outward, filling her lungs
with the pollen of freedom,
a future wider
than the sickroom.

No doubt she shed tears
to see his legs stiffen,
but she knew
that beneath salt
was sun, and sweetness,
and after mourning, joy.

As I cringe to see
my mother teeter,
each small sip an effort,
I try not to think
of the probable spring
in Gregor's sister's step
as she bleached his sheets.

Yet I imagine the sequence --
from sadness,
through relief,
to the intoxicating whiff
of the first brisk wind.

Focal Lengths

My mother looks at me
quite seriously. "It's all
an act," she says. "Why
do I have to be part of this?"
And I don't know whether
she means my joviality is an act,
or my reassurance, or whether
she herself, in continuing to place
foot before foot, knows
herself on stage, the curtain
near. Sometimes,

my lens is long enough
so that, focus clear,
I know it hopeless –
the massive vitamin
infusions, the hip and knee
massage, the biking
ordeal every day.

But with a macro lens,
and when she giggles
like a girl and kisses me,
it's a play I'm glad
to be cast in.

Lacking Memory...

Maybe
it's like waking from a dream
you feel shrouded within
before you've reached for,
tried to name, actually touched.
Details fade, till what's left
is the tongue's film of candy
sucked, or the damp coat
on hands quickly dried.

Maybe it's like lying on a bluff
where the sand near your feet
falls away. Though you scramble,
ground crumbles,
leaving nothing in place.

Maybe it's like driving at night
in the rain. Your eyes strain,
But signs pass too quickly
to read.

Your mind
can't get hands
to tell wheels
where to steer.

Maybe that's
how it feels.

The Gambler

Hunched over her bingo card,
you might expect to see
a cigarette in her mouth,
vodka in her bejeweled hand,
lipstick rings on napkins
near her nervous fingers.

But no, it is my plain-dressing,
clean living, demented mother
suddenly intent on winning
yet another prize, the first two
dime-store necklaces
vividly splayed on her chest,
she preening like some goddess
when I come for her.

"You can leave," she says sharply,
though she has no other
way home. "This is
a serious game."

Being of Use

I need onions.

My mother perks up.
"I think I have some,"
she says, and rises,
slow, but purposeful
as unlocking a door,
or carrying out the trash.

And in her search, perhaps
she travels into kitchens
full of children doing homework
round a table
while my father
reads the news.

She walks
through every room,
and comes back
carrying the cordless phone.
"Is this why I went?"
she asks,

        an onion drawing tears,
        its core near empty.

Of Art and Healing

Those clubbed nails
hugging my mother's toes
tightly as a baby's fist,
split, twisted as cardboard
curled by heat –

that ooze comes from fungus,
and will be killed with this
walnut tincture I apply.

Within three days, the skin
is dry, cuticles discrete.

Rimming each nail
is a smudge as black
as soil on the hands
of gardeners, paint
on the palms of artists
who use oils, charcoal
on cartoonist's fingers,
clay on sculptor's thumbs –

any of which I am,
as I whittle and shape
these live changing things.

What I Miss

After an award,
a triumph, the return
from a trip, I'd call,
knowing she'd gush,
full of questions.

The impulse remains.
I reach for the phone
to speak with my brass-band,
anxiety-riven mother,
her voice swiss-cheese rich
and riddled with love --

only to remember
she is now here with me,
perhaps even sitting
quite near, devolved

and child-like, a water color
running tears as she quavers,
"What next? "What day?"
"Where?"

Life's Rhythmic Relief

Some feel scant pressure
during life's daily story.
Young, elastic, not addicted
to tea or coffee, moderate
in habits, they act for a chapter
without interruption.

Most feel the urge more often –
once a page perhaps,
and can follow description,
enjoy dialogue,
take leisurely detours
around subject or task
before release. Older folks

might feel the need
every paragraph or two,
continuity more difficult,
more life spent in the loo,
zipping and unzipping, pulling up
or down, tearing paper
rolls away. But for my mom,

peeing comes between clauses,
which clutters thought
so as to almost obscure it,
itself co-subject,

so that ideas are dealt
like quick cards
between the long business
of discharge. The daily story

is thus broken, a shattered
mirror, each shard reflecting
discontinuous reality. Urgency
itself then gives meaning
to the passing of days:
life's rhythmic relief.

Ill-Prepared

When young, I was given
a round-bottomed doll.

I would pelt and pummel
its sloping sides,
giggling at its stubborn
stance, not able

to foresee how vital
robust balance would be,
or that I'd someday
clasp my lurching mother,
the world aswim for her,
the floor a roiling sea,

my self the solid prop
on which she leans.

The Stance

Arms up
against the door frame,
I have her push, pulling
shoulders back.
I press against
her spine as it grows
almost straight.

"See? I say.
"You don't have to stoop."

      "I do," she says,
head turned away.
"Because that's how I feel.
Diminished. I've lost
so much capacity,
I try to hide."

So we mourn
drained force, consider
others' pain, thank
for what remains.

"You're lucky,"
I say. "Stand straight."
And for a moment,
she does.

2007

Payoff

As my mother now
plies spoon or fork
to lift pills to her mouth,
I slip them through
her lips, then prompt
a drink.

It's like feeding
quarters at the laundry --
five or six till lights dim
and the water fills,
my thumb and fingers
stuffing a slit --

or thrusting pennies
through a piggie's hips.

In Las Vegas,
you pile coins in,
pull the lever
and pray. But here,
jackpots endure:

a functioning bowel, a heart
beating soundly, eyes
that open each morning,
aware.

Chantal's Pie

To my mother, the pie slice
was thrilling, its pears
and figs jagged, its prunes
the rocks of a terrain
she longed to climb.

But she found
she could not even
touch, could not bear to
break or have me cut,
it was so wild a trip
just to see, and so

she mimed a shrouding,
draped an open napkin
over the plate
to tame and put
imposing nature to bed,

at peace only

after I wrapped it
to be saved for a day
when scaling cliffs
was a skill
she might regain...

The Elements

In some ways similar,
she is water, I am air.

Her hyperbole feeds
my dramatic flair,
my love of the absurd
grown fat on her cackle.

When the pocketbook
I just held disappears,
neither under nor over,
up or around,
I too feel jaw clamp,
heart pound, a clenching
of the gut.

My bladder has also dropped.
Even by the jaunty
single hair -- white, curled,
proudly flying from the ends
of our chins -- we are linked.

But it is too much.
I swim in mother stuff,
and the damp breeds fungus.
I wheeze. And when the slog
is slow, as lung and brain
sip, I long for solitude: firm
    earth, clear
        skies, crisp
           air.

The First to Know

I didn't think she'd mind.
I'd had those tests
several times -- moving
tunnels, clanks, insect drones.

But they had to restrain
my mother with belts, and redo
shots. Dry mouthed and shaking,

she felt betrayed: How could
I let them experiment? For what?
She loathed x-rays,
from which she feared
slow death, and longed
to know whom to sue.

When I tried to explain –
days of dizziness, an arm
grown weak, slurred speech –
she was even more outraged.

"Don't you think I'd be
the first to know," she cried,
"if I'd had a stroke?"

Pomegranate Seeds

Luckily, my mother's
transient ischemic accident
was no worse than a pin
piercing the skin of a pomegranate.

Some little seeds burst, releasing
packets of linguistic category
that perhaps were always too rigid,
and are no worse for bleeding
the rich fluid of possibility.

So, when I forgot
to buy Depends,
and was distraught

she tried to comfort me.
"*Don't,*" she said, putting her
arm around my anguished
shoulders. "*Don't.... Don't....*"

And all the words to be found
in those delicate packets
migrated, then merged
to form a warm, juicy
command. "*Don't
besearch yourself,*" she said.

So I didn't.

Toileting

I don't know
whether she sought to read
a thermometer measuring
her own health,
or gauge the mercury
of my status, my function.
Perhaps she was just curious.

But in the midst
of a routine toilet- wash,
my mother stopped my hand,
alert and curious as a puppy
awaiting instruction, but with
a faint blush, a modesty,

as though suddenly aware
that it wasn't a usual
activity we were engaged in,
though I'd done it for years.

Do you," she asked,
and laughed a little bit,
perhaps sheepish --
"Do you do this
            for everyone?"

Systemic Crack

Quiet, resigned,
my incontinent mother
sits. Tubes between her legs
lead to a plastic bag below,
a camera- wand inside her.

On the monitor,
her bladder walls look clean:
honeycombed, the muscles
patterned as a latticed,
woven basket.

Often, swirls of liquid
surge like moving
clouds -- a flurry and swish
soon diffused as kidneys
add to the storage bank
of waste with the inevitability
of a waterfall,
or the persistent tide.

But somehow, these streams
tickle neurons
which induce my mother
to mindlessly release.

So a tiny flaw
along the line
cracks the system's
seamless binding.

The Elevator

When, after illness, the doors
spring apart, my mother's eyes
crackle fire. "When do you sleep?"
she marvels, though
it is only eight.

She is not sure
about the dining room.
"Is eating allowed this late?"

"What if they find us?"
she asks, as I pet her,
brush her hair, strew
our path with laughter.
"Do you have this much fun
with everyone?" she asks.

But when the door shuts,
her look stops seeing.
She can't find the sink
to spit in, the toilet to pee.
She holds the quilt
over her face, silent.

As it descends,
doors still open
on a floor. But each
stay is shorter

A Door with a Number

As in dreams,
her concept of place
is fluid. She floats
freely, now to a hut
with green trim, now
to a room full of lace –
fun, perhaps.
But as sites spin,
I sense fear
beneath her wonder.

Each time the bus
rolls her home
she is relieved
to find me, astonished
at the tire's magic turn,
mystified by the idea
of a house with a number
on the door.

She seems to believe
it a miracle – or perhaps
God's will, this bumbling
past millions of roosts
along a strange way
toward this best nest
where, calling for help,

someone loving always comes.

A Little Story

Although my mother
scorned toys,
I bought a cloth cat.
Lanky, not overstuffed,
it had silken hair
and a winsome face.

Months passed. My mother's
world blurred like an ink line
smears when wet. The cat,
with my aid, waved
and clapped. This
she came to accept.

Seeing him
nights before bed,
she named him, "Catsilah,"
and remembered his face.
His was the last good night kiss,
the final embrace.

It is a year. He brings her joy
she rarely gets from me.
His is the form imprinted
in a jumbled place.
When calm, he makes
her laugh. When afraid,
his presence quiets.

She speaks to him
in Yiddish, confiding
the news of the day.
Found in a thrift shop,
he cost fifty cents.

The Journey

When my mother
sucks on that straw, deeply,
there is a whirring sound,
like gears moving forward,
like spokes on the wagon
of my second grade primer,
Singing Wheels, rolling
across the prairie, having
adventures, achieving goals,
like the TGV speeding
through the French
countryside, getting
from Paris to Poitiers
tout de suite.

That prune juice
slipping down
my mother's throat
at great velocity, snaking
through her gut,
will find the optimal
drilling-spot,
et, voila, the result
will be as gratifying
as the trip.

Confessional Psalm

My mother is my shield.
I shall miss her protection.

She keeps me
from the offerings
of a tempting world.
Out of her need,
I weave a secret womb
for healing, wherein
there is peace

Yea, though I walk
past beckoning faces,
concerts, readings,
the wave of foreign flags,
I feel content here,

and treasure these solitary
years. Despite chores,
I often work in quiet,
my mother a zany model
who takes myriad poses
while I both kiss
and sketch, through which
we're both enriched.

Wild Fires

First the brush burns, the dry
under story, and then trees
flare, torches raging
against earth, sucking
air, glowing,

      And the firemen's jet
can tame the blaze to smoldering,
as do these drugs that I give my mother,
a constant manipulation of hosed
magic until all seems serene,
an innocent seething.

But beneath the skull,
ancient roots are eaten
like the wicks of bombs lit,

the fruit of ninety years
consumed by a licking,
orange crackle.

Shift / Change

Sometimes, now, her illness
is expressed as a simian grimace,
the lips pulled back to look
both menacing and mask-like.

Then her voice, perhaps
an octave below her norm,
croaks. Devoid of humor,
it is full of command
and the frustrated stutter
of incoherence.

This bark is not attractive,
and the mother I viewed
as an evolutionary jewel
now seems a pre-historic throw-back.

Somewhere, her spirit lives,
the body mere entrapment.

I can only mourn her absence,
and stand behind one of several shields:
an interest in medical pathology;
the concern of the anthropologist;

or the passion of a student
of chimps and great apes
in the forests of Africa.

That Home Song and Dance

She dons every sweater
she can sleeve into,
and then her coat, determined
to leave, this time for real.
Tired of being told
to bike, sick of the somehow
alien room, my mother's
out to find her real home.

"Let her go," says my husband
again. "Open the door.
I'll walk her down
so she won't trip." And as he

kisses her goodbye,
she suddenly wavers,
her eyes wide, mouth- lines
ironed, her face grown
young with the wonder of it.

When I am silent,
she sighs, pivots,
and "home" becomes a trip
upstairs again, a coat
unzipped, penitence.

But perhaps it is because
twenty minutes before
I'd slid half an Ativan
through her lips.

Sentient Beings

The hit cat drags itself
across the gutter, concrete
burning its wound like coals.
Even grass cuts.

The whale can't stand
the sonar squeal.
Bewildered, hungry
the white bear braves moving floes
as he tests impossible water.

And my mother's flesh
is trembling sinew,
eyes wild, clutch the grip
of the drowning, fingers
the feet of chickens
in my grandma's kitchen
half century ago,
yellow rope caked with scales.

When a string is tightened
past endurance,
it breaks, or the bridge
cracks, or the face
of the cello caves
and there's an end
to the music.

But with the suffering
of sentient beings
it is not so simple.

The Wanderer

That "wandering" they cite
in the Alzheimer texts
is no meander through
phlox, no stroll near ponds
on summer afternoons.

It is a 2 AM affair,
my mother determined
as a general in battle,
eyes flashing, hands
on any available sword.

She looks magnificent then:
cheeks ruddy with the enterprise,
shoulders thrown back farther
than I've seen in years,
she the eager form
on the prow of a ship
bound to fight the white whale.

As she struggles to dress,
indifferent to black- paned glass,
she needing only to leave, I see
both horse and jockey, intent
on the finish line, foam
on her lips. So,

her primal disease is intact --
that wild desire to get to,
arrive at, achieve.

The Need for Mother

"Does your back hurt?
she asks, after hours
of inert quiet,
as she sees me
straighten and groan.

Her small words
of maternal concern
will pop up sometimes,
like the tips of hosta emerging
from the stone-cold ground,
but with such insistent
warmth and caring
that one can imagine
the entire plant, live
and glowing green
beneath the earth.

This is what my sister
longed for, when she told
our mother of her daughter's
engagement -- this spark
from a past now almost
extinguished, which in memory
glows like a bonfire,
and makes her childhood
a sacred hearth.
For me, it was too rare
a gift to be relied on,
then. But I now gratefully
accept it.

Communicating with My Mother

My words chug through winding
tunnels, dimly lit and covered with dust,
cobwebs, gumballs, the litter
of long illness. I wait.

Often, there is wreckage,
the track uprooted.
At times an entire phrase
dies during travel. Sometimes,
it enters a crowded station
lined with moldy shelves
and shards of glass that clutter
the floor. This is the garbled
response center, and her reply
is a lump of guttural vowels
whose meaning you have to guess at.

But there are times
my questions find a high,
sun-filled room, the sofa
stylish, the curtains
bright and clean.

I remember her answers then --
speak of them.

Paeon to Geodon

If she fails to take
a small blue pill,
the desert spreads.

Grains of sand, inert,
bleached, know nothing
of the sun that beats.

If they speak,
their rasps stir weak
wheels in blazing heat.

They heave and roil
in their dry beds, their mouths
clamped shut.

Push in a pill, and wait
for strength to sputter,
spurt, and form
a plopping mud.

Then wrenching sobs
bathe a way
toward the world of the aware,

where neurons spark, and make
clean soil. Plants sprout, trees bud, then leaf.

This flowering is an ongoing gift
for my mother and me --
      a caregiver grateful for peace.

Becoming Accustomed

Anyone
who for years
saw her parents slip
sib night-soil
into toilets, then flush
to cleanse the yellow cloth,

learned
the process starts
with bottles boiled clean.
I'd watch my father's
open mouth
coax each bite
he fed each child.

Once you see
the flow of tides,
as water fills,
then leaves a cove,
or view cow flops,
doe's olive-pits,
the dung of dog,
bice goose-squirt strings—

you know the gut
a carousing artist
eager to try,
loath to repeat.

So, you'd forgive
any bowel-pranks
played in pre-dawn hours
in the silent house.

Vacancies

In my kitchen,
spent vitamin caps
lie on the counter
wantonly, each half
emptied of its power,
its powder poured
into the apple sauce
I feed my mother, as
"swallow" is no longer
understood.

Now, when left intact,
pills sit on her tongue
till dissolved, their contents
oozing down her chin
in lurid patterns, as shimmering
tattoos might mark some tribe
in Papua New Guinea.

So these small losses
gather, each diminution
echoing the void
in the fragments
I handle gently –

the nothing that is there,
and the nothing in my mother.

The Revelation

When we play bean bag,
I toss gently toward my mother's
chest, then watch her struggle –
not to catch, but to return
a pitch so that I'll never miss.

Intent on my success,
she almost places it
into my waiting hands.
I think it was terror
that we'd not succeed
that made her coax us so,
and put such force behind
each uphill thrust, there was
no way we'd fail
to earn the same high grades
next test.

There's been a cost –
four children who pull
life taut as they aim high.
But why?

For see how she smiles
when the game's not a test
but rather a gift; a clear space
where love is exchanged
as un-graded laughter:
a time for play.

Not Yet

You might think
I would have rid myself
of that old myth. The dead
are gone, beyond reach
or calling. But when,
ill for days, my mother
rises, looks at me
and calmly says, "It's time
to find my husband," the ice
that sometimes gathers near my heart
melts, flows over, floods. "We

don't know exactly where he is,"
she says, her voice
a luminous string
to which she clings
as she begins to tread
some fathomless bridge
that leads beyond my tears.

My caress pleads
with her eyes, now
grave, bright, and caught
in what seems
a moment of ultimate
seeing. Then I sculpt
my sobs to words,
and cast a net

that hauls her back, back--

promising she will of course
find him --- just
not yet.

Epilogue: The Next Step

When I tell her the plan,
my mother looks at me deeply.
We are as close
as lovers, our heads
on one pillow in the protective
dark. "When did you decide
to do this?" she asks. "Can I
back out?"

I hug her, hold her face
in my hands, say she'll probably
love it there. "After I try it,
will I have a choice?"
I nod, and our eyes
stroke one another slowly.
"But I like my life here," she says.

Time is a windy
accordion after she leaves,
its bellows torn and wheezing.
I feel a tug at what was
our common web and is now
merely air and a gnawing
stickiness seeking attachment.
The staff there says she
sometimes looks around
and shakes her head. "Maybe

she'll come back soon,"
they hear her say,
long after such patients
should forget. These words

catch, then cut my throat
as I bleed tears.

Glossary

Milk and Meat: *Shul* is a synagogue; *Shabos*, the Jewish
Sabbath; Moses received the prohibition against boiling a
kid in its mother's milk in tablets at Mt. Sinai. Exodus and
Deuteronomy.

Awareness: Seder is the Passover ritual meal; haroset is a
mixture, often of chopped apple, walnut, and wine, which
represents the mortar used by enslaved Jews in Egypt.
Afikomen is the middle matzo in a stack of three, meant
to be hidden by the youngest child present, then ransomed
comedically. Matzo is flat, unleavened bread eaten during
Passover.

What She Wants: *tsuzamen* is Yiddish for "together."

A Prayer to the Dial Tone: *davening* is Yiddish for a form of
praying which often involves movement.

Afterward

After the book was finished, the reconciliation such a care-giving situation can affect became clear to me. Old wounds had been healed through role-reversal. Touch, kindness, and humor, perhaps at first deliberate, but soon natural, eased our formerly tense relationship. Now in charge and loving, my past anger dissolved.

My mother's larger biography, which weds hard work to extensive study, anxiety, religious conflict, warm exuberance and passionate family involvement – will be illuminated in my next book, *Moving Stills: A Life in Stories*, now in search of a publisher. But much of my mother's late-life story lies outside the scope of the poems in *Not Yet*.

For several years before I "kidnapped" her, she lived alone in Brooklyn, my father long dead, she already suffering moderate dementia: stopping traffic with an outstretched umbrella, barging into random dentist's offices to demand treatment, filling her apartment with piles of old clothes. I phoned six times a day to encourage vitamins/meds.

During the time she lived with me, she went to a magnificent day-care center on Long Island, NY, aptly named "Day Haven." The director, Ethel Thomas, maximized functionality, maintained dignity, and infused each day with laughter. For my mother, the routine extended the rhythms of a work-filled life. Her abilities fluctuated erratically over these 3 ½ years, but she enjoyed her "school" throughout.

Then my sister Jessica found a fine live-in dementia accommodation in Aurora, Colorado. Called "Juniper Village," the care–givers were warm, efficient, emotionally invested. "Assisted living," the facility felt domestic rather than institutional. Mom lived here for another 3 ½ years. Jessica hired auxiliary help for her, and superintended her care.

Doris (Dora, to family) died December 4, 2010, on the fourth day of Chanukah—the day of my father's death thirty three years earlier. We like to think he came to get her. My sister and her family all remained with her at the end, throughout and after, coaching her the way one would a woman giving birth. And it was around this time that SFA Press accepted *Not Yet* for publication. Laura McKinney and Brittany O'Sullivan were the able editors/designers.

I thank all who read for me and made suggestions for revision: Carin Clevidence, Adele Glimm / Myriam Chapman's writing group in NY, Orel Protopopescu / Claire White's Stony Brook group, Cortney Davis, the exacting Trina Porte (Chickaree Press), Connie Smilowitz, and my longtime partner Dan Maciejak.

Cover photo of my mother, Doris Smilowitz (1927-2010), by Arthur Silk, www.silkphoto.com; cover design vanhowell@btopenworld.com, Van Howell; Thanks to jackdepietromusic@gmail.com and Paul Antonell, the Club House, Rhinebeck NY 12572, for the recorded CD. The CD was produced by DiscMakers, Pennsauken, NJ 08110. Thanks to Jenn Twarowski, Project Manager at DiskMakers.

Book Club Discussion

1. Did you get a clear idea of an evolving relationship by reading the 94 poems? What did you come away with by the book's end?

2. Which of the mother's personality traits come out clearly in the poems? What did you learn about the daughter during the course of the book? Explain.

3. How is illness handled throughout the book? What did you learn about Alzheimer's as a disease through these proems? What changes in the mother's physical and emotional state are evident during the four year period covered in the book?

4. What aspects of care-giving seem most stressful to the daughter/poet? What helps mitigate these strains? What does the daughter find nourishing about the care-giving relationship? How has the poet's attitude toward her mother changed?

5. Comment on the diverse focus of these poems. Pick five poems that seemed strangest, most bizarre. Discuss.

6. How do psych meds influence the mother's behavior and the daughter's reactions?

7. Were these poems accessible and easy to understand? How did the use of poetry enhance the telling of this story?

8. What role did 'adult day care' programs play in the life of an Alzheimer patient as shown in this book?

9. Dora comes from a Jewish family. How did the mention of cultural practices impact your experience of the book?

10. Pick five poems you really liked and explain why.

About the Author

Now retired from teaching, farming, and care-giving, Marcia Slatkin plays cello, does photo-collage, and writes fiction, drama, poetry. Two of her stories won **PEN** fiction prizes, 18 have been published in literary journals, most recently in *Gargoyle*, *Lilith*, and *Midstream*. 16 of her one-act plays have been produced in off-off Broadway theatres; one of her full lengths, *Upside Down*, won a staged reading at the **Long Beach Theater**, CA in 2010 and six non-equity performances produced by Tony White in NYC in 2011. Finalist in the *Barnyard Women Poets*, the *John Ciardi*, and the *Context Magazine* contests, her poems have been published in journals like *The Paris Review*, *Crone*, *Xanadu*, and *Calyx*. Her full length collection, *A Woman Milking: Barnyard Poems*, was published by **Word Press** in 2006. Her two beautiful, intelligent, interesting daughters grown, she now lives with her partner Dan, with whom she travels, and cultivates gardens. Please see www.marciaslatkin.com